# YOUR KNOWLEDGE HAS VALUE

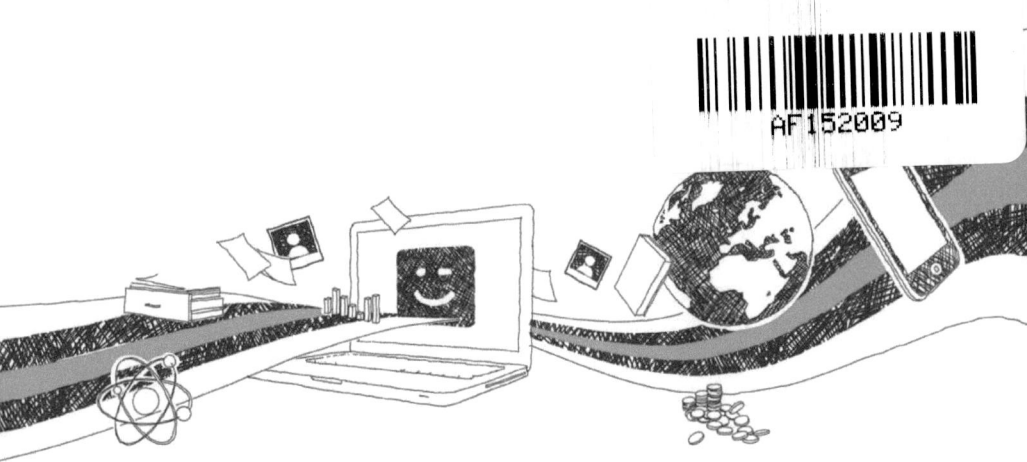
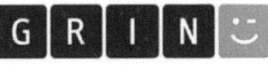

Kim Wong

# Managing and consequences of physician to patient ratio in health care organizations

GRIN Publishing

**Imprint:**

Copyright © 2012 GRIN Verlag GmbH
Print and binding: Books on Demand GmbH, Norderstedt Germany
ISBN: 978-3-656-82384-1

**This book at GRIN:**

http://www.grin.com/en/e-book/283072/managing-and-consequences-of-physician-to-patient-ratio-in-health-care

**GRIN - Your knowledge has value**

Since its foundation in 1998, GRIN has specialized in publishing academic texts by students, college teachers and other academics as e-book and printed book. The website www.grin.com is an ideal platform for presenting term papers, final papers, scientific essays, dissertations and specialist books.

**Visit us on the internet:**

http://www.grin.com/

http://www.facebook.com/grincom

http://www.twitter.com/grin_com

Vor- und Nachname   Yanbo.Wang

Thema der Masterarbeit

Managing and consequences of physician to patient ratio in health care

organizations

Masterarbeit im Fach  Management in der Medizin

Vorgelegt in der Masterprüfung

im Studiengang Medizinökonomie

der Wirtschafts- und Sozialwissenschaftlichen Fakultät der Universität zu Köln

Prüfungsamt für Gesundheitsökonomie

Universität zu Köln

Ort, Datum   Köln   26.11.2012

# Table of Contents

# Key Acronyms

| FTE | Full Time Equivalent |
|-----|----------------------|
| GDP | Gross Domestic Product |
| GME | Graduate Medical Education |
| NP | Nurse Practitioner |
| NPC | Non-Physician Clinician |
| PA | Physician Assistant |
| PC | Primary Care |

## List of Exhibits

# 1. Introduction

Imbalance between demand for and supply of physicians is an issue regularly addressed by the media, researchers and policy makers. It has been widely spread in many countries for years. Healthcare organizations in both of developed and developing countries have all experienced from that. Physician to patient ratio is one of the important normative population based indicators to measure this imbalance. It equals to the entire number of physicians in a healthcare organization dividing its patient volume within a certain period (e.g., a year). The quotient is often standardized in form of X (number of physicians) per 1,000 patients, or in form of "1:X" in order to express the amount of patients (X) that under one physician's management clearly. In comparison with other measurements, this kind of indicators are less complicated and easier to comprehend. An imbalance between physician demand and supply in a healthcare organization could be explicitly identified and quantified by comparing its actual physician to patient ratio with a "gold standard".[1] Unfortunately, a wide-range suitable gold standard of physician to patient ratio does not exist. Therefore, healthcare organizations must make great efforts to find their own gold standards.

The physician to patient ratio could be easily confounded with the patient to physician ratio which represents the number of physicians, who oversee one patient within his or her entire hospital stay. In an ideal model for patient care is "1:1" the target patient to physician ratio to aim at. But in reality, this ratio is not easy to realize.[2] In this paper, merely the physician to patient ratio is under discussion.

Imbalance between demand for and supply of physicians could bring inappropriate physician to patient ratio to healthcare organizations. It is one of the major threats to healthcare organizations, as it might have consequences such as lower quality of healthcare services, closure of hospital's ward, increasing wait time, reducing number of staff beds, under-utilization of physicians or higher medical costs.[3] Managing the physician to patient ratio is not only a key to predict these risks but also the hope for turning the imbalance situations into balance

---

1. Zurn et al. 2002, P. 39
2. Hospitalist management advisor 2008, P. 6
3. Zurn et al. 2002, P. 1

ones.

Finding the right physician to patient ratio (gold standard) and realizing it should be ranked as a significant issue facing healthcare organizations, since it is essential for achieving high efficiencies. And this mission seems to be much more important and difficult in an era of physician shortage than physician surplus.

In the first section of this paper, the possible consequences for healthcare organizations related to physician to patient ratio of different categories are considered. The factors that affect the physician to patient ratio are presented in the second section. Finally, the third section, offers an introduction and analysis of the methods and techniques for finding and realizing the right physician to patient ratio in healthcare organizations.

## 2. Consequences of physician to patient ratio in healthcare organizations

The selected gold standard physician to patient ratio of a healthcare organization is the benchmark to evaluate its actual physician to patient ratio. The "gold standard" itself should be the most appropriate ratio for the healthcare organization. In terms of the complexity of the reality, even the "gold standard" is founded, it is often difficult to achieve. The actual physician to patient ratio of a healthcare organization around its "gold standard" (not too low or too high) is thus also appropriate for it. The physician to patient ratio can reflect the status of balance between physician demand and supply within a healthcare organization. Only the lower or higher than appropriate (excessively low or high) ratio could break the balance status and arise various of problems. The physician to patient ratio could respectively be observed from managerial perspective (e.g., ratio of an ICU in a hospital) and system perspective (e.g. ratio of a region), and thus its related consequences. Before discussion of the consequences, some statistics about physician to patient ratio from empirical studies are exhibited following.

The interdisciplinary operative intensive care unit of university hospital Jena has 14 physicians (4 chef physicians, 10 assistant physicians). They treated 3,773 patients in 2010. In other words, the physician to patient ratio of this ICU in 2010 is approximately 1:270.[1] (Observation from managerial perspective)

---

1. Riedemann et al. 2012, w.p. (without page)

**Exhibit 1. Physician to patient ratio of some regions in the USA**

(Observation from system perspective)

| COUNTY | STATE | DOCTORS PER 10,000 (2006) |
|--------|-------|---------------------------|
| DeKalb | AL | 5.74 |
| Jackson | AL | 9.76 |
| Bartow | GA | 13.14 |
| Catoosa | GA | 22.59 |
| Chattooga | GA | 4.63 |
| Dade | GA | 11.33 |
| Fannin | GA | 17.45 |
| Floyd | GA | 32.57 |
| Gilmer | GA | 9.54 |
| Gordon | GA | 11.88 |
| Murray | GA | 4.23 |
| Pickens | GA | 10.65 |
| Walker | GA | 4.9 |
| Whitfield | GA | 20.88 |
| Cherokee | NC | 14.2 |

Note: AL - Alabama Georgia, GA - Georgia, NC - North Carolina
Source: Alabama Board of Medical Examiners, Georgia Board for Physician Workforce,
North Carolina Health Professions Data System

The above exhibit clearly indicates that the physician to patient ratio can vary a lot from region to region, even in the USA.

## 2.1 Outcomes of appropriate physician to patient ratio

An adequate physician supply of a healthcare organization has specialty, geographic, and time dimensions. In other words, it could be defined as "having the right number of physicians, with the right skills, in the right place, at the right time".[1] An adequate physician supply is always required from a healthcare organization to help ensure access to affordable, quality healthcare, as it can contribute to appropriate physician to patient ratio.[2]

---

1. Council of state Governments 2008, P. 2
2. Bureau of health professions et al. 2008, P. 4

## Observation from managerial perspective

Running with an appropriate physician to patient ratio could imply to a healthcare organization that, it has sufficient physicians to treat the entire patients with high quality medical services, and simultaneously each physician has the possibility to enjoy the balance between work and family life. In this situation the physicians will not overwork or be occupied with nothing. Besides, they could also get opportunities and enough time to engage in advanced studies or trainings. A timely update of medical knowledge and techniques is essential for a physician's career life.

## Observation from system perspective

For various participants in healthcare system such as physicians, patients, insurers, non-physician clinicians (NPCs) the expected consequences of an appropriate physician to patient ratio could be quite different.

From a physician perspective, the consequence of an appropriate physician to patient ratio is that a healthcare organization is capable to ensure all of its patients accessing to quality care, but the physicians supply of this organization should never be so large that it induces excessive competition for the existing patient base. Physician earnings will decrease when too many physicians competing for a limited number of insurance contacts.[1]

From a patient perspective, a healthcare organization with an appropriate physician to patient ratio is where he/she can receive prompt and high-quality healthcare services. Economic considerations such as inefficiencies created by an oversupply of physicians are lesser important for most patients who are shielded from the entire direct cost of care.[1]

From an insurer's perspective, the consequence of an appropriate physician to patient ratio is that a healthcare organization provides a socially acceptable level of healthcare services for a minimum cost.[1]

From a NPC's perspective, the consequence of an appropriate physician to patients ratio is that a hospital could not only ensure adequate delivery of quality

---

1. Bureau of health professions et al. 2008, P. 63

healthcare, but also could supply sufficient employment opportunities for them.[1] Experienced NPCs such as NPs (Nurse Practitioners) and PAs (Physician Assistants) can do the same job as physicians for a fraction of the cost, so the utilization of these workforce could extensively reduce the personnel costs.[2]

From society's perspective, healthcare should be provided in the most-effective manner. So when a healthcare organization ensure patient access to quality healthcare with an appropriate physician to patient ratio, significant inefficiencies should not be created, even some of them such as having sufficient physician workforce to handle unexpected surges in healthcare demand are acceptable from a societal perspective.[3]

## 2.2 Outcomes of inappropriate physician to patient ratio

A physician shortage/surplus is the result of a disequilibrium between the demand for and supply of physician workforce. It is a major factor that could bring inappropriate (lower or higher than appropriate) physician to patient ratio to healthcare organizations. Physician shortage is an enormous threat to healthcare organizations. When the patients in a healthcare organization are too many to handle, consequences such as lower quality of health services, loss of productivity, increasing wait time and length of stay, decreasing patient satisfaction, and under-utilization of   might occur.[4] Under the threats of a severe physician shortage caused excessively low physician to patient ratio, healthcare organizations could usually not keep the promise of being open at their full capacity to care for its communities. Insufficient number and mix of personnel to care for patients compels them to reduce access to healthcare, including reducing the number of staff beds and postponing or cancelling elective surgeries.[5] On the contrary, a surplus of physicians is less dangerous. When the physician workforce of a healthcare organization is sufficient for its healthcare delivery and simultaneously some of them sit idly in their working time, problems such as higher medical spending, increasing unnecessary medical procedures might arise. The focus of

---

1. Bureau of health professions et al. 2008, P. 63
2. Dark 2011, w.p.
3. Bureau of health professions et al. 2008, P. 62
4. Zurn et al. 2002, P. 1; Hospitalist management advisor 2008, P. 1
5. Iroquois healthcare alliance 2008, P. 1

the following two parts of this section is oriented towards a detailed presentation and analysis of the consequences of inappropriate physician to patient ratio in healthcare organizations.

## 2.2.1 Outcomes of lower than appropriate physician to patient ratio

Shortage is a relative notion.[1] A physician shortage in an European healthcare organization would probably be viewed as a physician surplus from an African perspective. Therefore, being aware of the context of a healthcare organization is important for assessing the balance status between its demand for and supply of physician labor.

### Observation from managerial perspective

Physician shortage based lower than appropriate physician to patient ratio is undesirable, since a physician shortage places heavy burden on physicians to treat larger patient loads.[2] Healthcare organizations should not care more patients than they can manage. If the patients are too many to handle, the excess demand will result in a never-ending and ever-expanding delay in service delivery in addition to bump the patients to other providers, resulting in discontinuity.[3] When a physician tries to see more patients each day, he or she has to cut back an time with every patient or glosses over them superficially, which may cause things to get missed or raise the chance of errors (e.g., make a mistake when writing prescriptions).[4] Physician overwork could decrease the quality of healthcare, increase the length of stay and finally resulting in lower insurance reimbursement. In addition, the possibilities that morbidities and mortality raises, long-term costs skyrocket will be much higher in healthcare organizations.[5]

Longer wait times for patients to schedule an appointment with a healthcare organization and to arrive at a scheduled appointment are two important indicators of a lower than appropriate physician to patient ratio. The number of patients a

1. Zurn et al. 2002, P. 1
2. Bureau of health professions et al. 2008, P. 63
3. Murray et al. 2007, P. 46
4. Hospitalist management advisor 2008, P. 1; Noton 2009, w.p.
5. Hospitalist management advisor 2008, P. 1

healthcare organization can effectively care for always has a limit. If an organization keeps saying "yes" to new patients and exceeds that limit, the overload can initially be absorbed into patients waiting time. Unfortunately, patients' patience of waiting also has a limit. They will quit at some point. Besides, the increasing waiting times for an appointments can induce escalating chaos within a healthcare organization evidenced by an increased number of phone calls; longer time to handle those calls; more patient complaints; increasing no-show, cancel and reschedule rates; greater utilization of triage resources to determine who has to wait and who cannot wait; and an increased degree of discontinuity, which harms patient outcomes and satisfaction and raises the return visit rate and length of visit, which in turn decreases productivity.[1]

In the USA, the average wait time for new patients to schedule an appointment with all physician specialties was relatively constant during the early-to-mid 1990s, but increased in the late 1990s and early 2000s.[2] In mainland china, in Jiangsu provincial hospital (first affiliated hospital of Nanjing medical university), the waiting passages outside almost all its specialties are often fulfilled with patients. Since the patient base in Jiangsu province is enormous and the system of referral never exists in this country, there is no appointment between new patients and hospitals. New patients come directly to the hospital, register themselves and visit the physicians according to the order of their registrations. The average wait time for them to visit a physician is on average at least 45 minutes and the time a physician sees a patient is maximum five minutes in this hospital. The register quantity of every specialty particularly of some prestigious specialists is limited for the patients every half day. In order to get the opportunity to visit a famous specialist, some patients wait already for registration before the hospital opens, even in the cold winter morning. Although this "first register first server" model has many shortcomings, but when a patient is early enough, he or she can visit the physician within a half day. Patients in Germany at least in Wurzburg and cologne could often wait more than two weeks to visit a specialist.

1. Murray 2007, P. 49-50
2. Bureau of health professions et al. 2008, P. 63

## Observation from system perspective

A lower than appropriate physician to patient ratio is always accompanied by raised physician income and improved choice of employment opportunities. While the improved choice of employment opportunities signals the demand for more physicians, raised physician income offers the economic incentives to enter the medical profession, to reallocate to a particular residency and to delay retirement.[1]

Competition among physicians could strengthen the insurer's hand in negotiating payment discounts. Hence insurers are not willing to undergo a physician shortage based lower than appropriate physician to patient ratio, as too few physicians will limit this competition, drives up recruiting and labor costs, and drives down the sale value of existing physician practices.[2]

The physician workforce of healthcare organizations influences not only the health status of local communities but also the economy of a local population or state as well. As employers, purchasers, and residents, they are vital to the economy. "Directly, physicians create and support jobs; purchase products and services; generate revenue to state/local governments; help develop new industries and businesses; help attract new residents; and contribute to local hospitals through inpatient admissions and outpatient services, and to larger health systems through referrals. Indirectly, physicians lend to a community's increased household spending and greater economic activity." It is estimated that the direct economic impact of a specialist in New Jersey is $3,000,000 per year and the total economic impact annually is $4,517,727. This implicates that the undersupply of each specialist can decrease the household income of a community there by $4.5 million. It is estimated that the total financial loss of New Jersey owing to (all kinds of) physician shortage is over $5.6 billion in 2010.[3]

All in all, a physician shortage based lower than appropriate physician to patient ratio threats not only the healthcare organizations, but also the whole society. Strategies and policies for physician workforce management must be updated in time to avoid the physician shortage and its associated consequences. A less than appropriate physician to patient ratio should never be forgotten as warning signal

---

1. Bureau of health professions et al. 2008,  P. 65-66
2. Bureau of health professions et al. 2008,  P. 68
3. New Jersey Council of Teaching Hospitals 2010, P. 1-2

of a physician undersupply in healthcare organizations.

## 2.2.2 Outcomes of higher than appropriate physician to patient ratio

In contrast to physician shortfall, physician surplus is difficult to appear, since there are series of policies and programs which can effectively stop the physician supply from increasing. From the mid-1970s, some observers of the United States began to forecast physician surplus in their country.[1] Nevertheless, until recently, the relevant economic evidence of physician surpluses in the USA has still not emerged.[2] Although a physician surplus is not easy to come up, being aware of the consequences of a physician surplus based higher than appropriate physician to patient ratio in healthcare organizations should never be ignored.

### Observation from system perspective

In a competitive market, a physician surplus based higher than appropriate physician to patient ratio would be assumed to result in a fall of the physician earnings and decreased choices of employment opportunities. Between 1990 and 2000, hourly earnings of the American physicians declined by 5 percent on average. Surgical specialties and obstetrics and gynecology have experienced the largest decline among all of the physicians during those years. Their mean hourly earnings reduced respectively by 14.1 and 13.7 percent.[3]

In an era of physician oversupply, a higher than appropriate physician to patients ratio allows a healthcare organization to be more selective in hiring physicians. Fewer employment opportunities, longer wait time to find a employment , less satisfied starting salary and location are typical problems for the new physicians graduates to confront in such a time. A 1996 survey of graduating residents and fellows of America in internal medicine showed that, 53% of them in infectious diseases faced with significant difficulties in receiving a practice position and 29% received only one job offer. In contrast, finding a practice location is much easier for the new physician graduates in general internal

---

1. Zurn et al. 2002, P. 25
2. Dill/Salsberg 2008, P. 13
3. Bureau of health professions et al. 2008, P. 66

medicine. Only 23% of them indicated significant difficulty and only 12% received only one job offer.[1]

Besides the above mentioned two consequences, other possible outcomes of a physician surplus (shortage) based higher (lower) than appropriate physician to patient ratio are summarized in Exhibit 2. The following table could be seen as a summary for the last two parts (1.2.1 and 1.2.2) of this section.

**Exhibit 2. Consequences of an inappropriate physician to patients ratio**

| Outcome category | Outcomes of a higher (lower) than appropriate physician to patient ratio |
|---|---|
| Observation from system perspective | 1. Mean hourly earnings of physicians are lower (higher) than expected earnings<br>2. Less (more) employment opportunities for new physicians<br>3. The price of healthcare services fluctuates downward (upward)<br>4. Insures have more (less) selections in hiring physicians<br>6. Physicians are more (less) interested in relocating<br>7. Physicians are more (less) interested in changing specialty<br>8. NPCs have greater (fewer) problems obtaining employment |
| Observation from managerial perspective | 1. Accessibility, continuity and quality of care of healthcare organization for individuals is lower (higher)<br>2. Wait times for patients at physician's offices are shorter (longer)<br>3. Wait times in scheduling appointments for patients (especially new patients) are shorter (longer)<br>4. The average length of waiting between patient follow-up visits reduces (rises)<br>5. Compared to historical standards individual physicians see fewer (more) patients hourly<br>6. Individual physicians work shorter (longer) daily<br>7. The retirement of physicians is earlier (delayed)<br>8. More (less) healthcare services with marginal medical value are delivered by physicians |

Source: Bureau of health professions et al. 2008, P.65 and self rewrite

The above elements do not represent an exhaustive consequences list of inappropriate physician to patient ratio. All of these Consequences could also be

---

1. Bureau of health professions et al. 2008, P. 67

treated as indicators of a physician surplus/shortage and an imbalance between demand for and supply of physicians in healthcare organizations.

### 3. Factors affecting physician to patient ratio

A successful management of physician to patient ratio in healthcare organizations is based on a good understanding of the factors affecting it and their affecting mechanisms. Factors often influence physician to patient ratio in healthcare organizations via increasing/decreasing their physician demand/supply. While economic and population trends drive the demand for physicians, work effort of physician and physician productivity are typical elements that could determine the supply of physicians. These factors could thus also be defined as determinants of physician demand or supply. They could simply be divided into two groups, namely system level and managerial level determinants.

### 3.1 Determinants of physician demand
### 3.1.1 Determinants of physician demand in system level

#### Economy

Economy is the major trend that affects the demand for physician services. In most of the developed countries, healthcare costs has been closely attached to levels of economic development, as reflected by the per capita gross domestic product (GDP) of a country.[1] Both theory and empirical evidence have proved that there exists a positive correlation between GDP and demand for physician workforce.[2] The ability and willingness to pay for physician services increases in pace with the growth of the economic wellbeing.[3] Cooper and others have explored that the physician to population ratio (a supply measure used as a proxy for demand) increases by 0.75% for each 1% increase in per capital GDP.[4] Since physician to patient ratio in healthcare organizations often changes with physician to population ratio together, the former would also increase in terms of the

---

1. Getzen 2000, P. 66
2. Cooper et al. 2012, P. 143
3. Dill/Salsberg 2008, P. 50
4. Cooper et al. 2012, P. 145

economic expansion. Hence we could suppose that there's also a correlation between physician to patient ratio in healthcare organizations and GDP. If this relationship really exists, three important points must be considered in interpreting it.

First, the sensitivity to economic wellbeing of different specialties could vary a lot. For instance, specialties delivering significant amounts of elective care (e.g., plastic surgeons) are likely more sensitive to economy than specialties providing less elective care (e.g., internist).[1] Thus, it is not a surprise that while each 1% increase in GDP drives up the demand for plastic surgery by 1% (elasticity=1.0), only 0.25% more general internal medicine is required.

Second, the slope (e.g., 0.75:1) of this mathematical correlation is not constant. It is a long-term macrotrend. Microturbulence such as governmental regulation or changes in the structure of health plans may lead to deviations, but only within a relative short period of time.[2]

Finally, the relationship between GDP and the demand for physician services is the consequence of countervailing societal factors that both promote and constrain physician use. Efforts to increase the healthcare spending are always balanced by reforms that aim at constraining costs and limit access. Even so, physician demand could also deviate far from its long-term relationship with GDP infrequently.

**Demographic trends**

Population growth and aging are two major demographic trends that affect the physician demand in healthcare organizations. While population growth could drive the overall demand for physician services upward, population aging may sharply increase the demand for specialties (e.g., cardiologists) that predominantly serve the elderly.[3]

It is estimated that more than 51.2 million (to 349.4 million) population will increase in the US between 2006 and 2025, with the elderly (65+ population) constituting more than a half of this growth (26.3 million). It implicates that the

---

1. Dill/Salsberg 2008, P. 51
2. Cooper et al. 2012, P. 145
3. Dill/Salsberg 2008, P. 7

elderly will increase obviously faster than the non-elderly. Furthermore, the population age 75 and older (the oldest segment) is forecasted to grow fastest with a percentage of 52%.[1] The 51.2 million population alone could lead to an enormous growth in the demand for physician workforce. An aging population will assure this growth.[2]

Many diseases are more prevalent among the elderly population. As the 65+ population increases, many disorders especially chronic conditions are likely to spread with a rapidity in this age group. As medical science and techniques continue to improve, this could mean that the elderly will live longer with multi-morbidities and thus require more intensive and sustained healthcare services.[3]

The elderly consumes twice as many physician services as the non-elderly. In 2006, there were approximately 18.3 million 75+ population in the US (approximately 6% of the total US population), but they used 17% of the entire physician hours. By 2030, the number of the 65+ population in the US will be more than 71 million, which is twice as many as their number in 2000.[4] Most of the growth in demand from the elderly could be attributable to the growth in their sheer numbers, rather than the shift in the age structure of the population.[5]

The major demographic trends in Germany are depopulation and population aging. After 2020 the population in Germany would first slowly, then rapidly decrease. It is forecasted that approximately 4.6 Million population will decrease in Germany between 2012 and 2040.[6] However, demand for physician services in German healthcare organizations could also be expected to increase in terms of other important factors (e.g. doubled aging).

### 3.1.2 Determinants of physician demand in managerial level

#### NPC workforce

NPCs' provision of "physician services" is an important factor that could decrease the physician demand in healthcare organizations. The restrictions of NPCs'

1. Dill/Salsberg 2008, P. 42
2. Dill/Salsberg 2008, P. 28
3. Institute of medicine of the national academies 2008, P. 1; Salsberg/Grover 2006, P. 783
4. Dill/Salsberg 2008, P. 13
5. Dill/Salsberg 2008, P. 20
6. Rürup 2003, P. 54-55

potential to substitute for physicians are their authorized prerogatives and their entire number, but in the US both of these restrictions are diminishing now. The substitution function of NPCs is substantial, as most of them now deliver not only adjunctive services but also services that broadly overlap those delivered by physicians. Their numbers are also increasing. It is predicted that by 2015 there are as many as 525,000 NPCs engaged in primary care and specific specialties in the US. Their combined output will be equivalent to approximately 65 physicians serving 100,000 population. Most of this increase will be focused on primary care, which has a relatively stable demand for NPCs. However, the fastest growth of demand for physician workforce is in the non-primary care specialties, to which NPCs devote generally proportionately less.[1] Hence healthcare organization such as primary care center should make better use of NPCs than other kinds of healthcare organizations (e.g., hospital).

**Gender**

The physician services utilization of female are quite different from males. Despite of the earliest years of life, far more physician services for women than for men are required. Women often need more physician services in the surgery and other specialties such as neurology, pathology, and radiology especially from 18 to 44 years. Among those 75 years of age and older, women's requirement for primary care is much greater than men, since they usually live longer and comprise a larger percentage of the elderly than men do. As the population ages the large amount of elderly women will greatly impact the entirety of the healthcare delivery system.[2]

Owing to the gender differences in the utilization of physician services, healthcare organizations must take the gender composition of their patients into account when managing physician to patient ratio. Otherwise, even if the physician to patient ratio of a healthcare organization equals to its "gold standard", negative consequences could also arise.

---

1. Cooper et al. 2012, P. 147-148
2. Dill/Salsberg 2008, P. 31-32

## 3.2 Determinants of physician supply

### 3.2.1 Determinants of physician supply in system level

**New physician graduates**

Medical School Graduates are the fountain of physician supply. In the United States, approximately 24,000 medical students accomplish their training through Graduate medical education (GME) programs and become new physicians each year. They enter practice through one of three routes: completing a U.S. school of allopathic or osteopathic medicine, or completing an international medical school. U.S. allopathic medical schools devote in recent years approximately 15,000 to 16,000 graduates to their healthcare systems, which is at most among these three types of medical schools. The latter two sorts of medical schools could respectively contribute approximately 2400 and over 5000 new physicians each year.[1] Workforce of new physician graduates deserves the attention of healthcare organizations, since it is not only an essential element of the physician supply, but also the future of the entire healthcare industry.

**Choice of Specialty**

A good comprehension of new physician's specialty choice and its determinants should be of great interest for healthcare organizations. After graduation from medical schools, physicians have to choose their specialties and enter a residency program. Individual interest, ability, desired lifestyle, expected prestige and payment are all important physician internal factors that affect their choices. Available residency slot, policy and market factors such as perceived employment opportunities are external factors for new physicians that sometimes could restrict their career life.[2] It is noteworthy that the specialty choice of new physicians can determine the long-term physician supply of healthcare organizations.

---

1. Bureau of health professions et al. 2008, P. 9-10
2. Bureau of health professions et al. 2008, P. 12

### 3.2.2 Determinants of physician supply in managerial level

**Physician work effort**

Physician work effort is nowadays in the direction of reducing. Aging of the physicians (with its associated decrease in working hours), the increase of female physicians, the lesser work effort of employed physicians, the tendency of younger physicians to require more personal time, the incremental frequency of early retirement, and the digressive hours that residents tend to work are all important elements that could induce a rapid decrease of the physician supply in healthcare systems.[1]

**Physician productivity**

The overall supply of physician services could increase (decrease) on the basis of an increase (decrease) in physician productivity. Entire patient serving hours, number of patients treated or the revenue generated during a given period are often used to measure the productivity of physicians.[2] Although total working hours of the physicians in many developed countries are declining, it does not represent a loss of physician productivity in these countries. Improved science and technology, improved education, and increased efficiency in healthcare delivery are all powerful locomotives that promote the physician productivity continue to increase.[3] For healthcare organizations, a careful analysis of trends in physician productivity is the foundation of a successful projection of physician supply.

### 4. Management of physician to patient ratio in healthcare organizations

The difficulty of physician to patient ratio management differs regarding to the scale of healthcare organization, and thus also the management methodology. For small-scale management (e.g., managing the physician to patient ratio for an individual physician or practice), we should use "direct management methodology",

1. Cooper et al. 2012, P. 147
2. Bureau of health professions et al. 2008, P. 13
3. Bureau of health professions et al. 2008, P. 25

und for large healthcare organization such as hospital and clinic, "indirect management methodology". These two methodologies are concrete analyzed and discussed in this section.

## 4.1 Direct management methodology

The three steps to a successful small-scale management of physician to patient ratio should be finding a gold standard of physician to patient ratio, defining the current ratio and comparing it with the gold standard, and adjusting and improving the actual ratio. The managing procedure is in this part proposed.

The number of patients a physician can effectively care for is limited. It must be defined, since it is significant for healthcare organizations to manage clinical workloads and optimize access to care of patients. This limit depends on myriad factors but mainly on the healthcare system in which he/she practices.[1] Hence the appropriate physician to patient ratio could vary a lot from physician to physician, from healthcare organization to healthcare organization, from region to region... Since the small-scale management of physician to patient ratio in the field of primary care (PC) is relative easier than in the other fields of healthcare, I set it as the starting line of understanding the management procedure.

"Panel size" is a key word in the field of PC. It is simply the number of individual patients (regularly) under the care of a specific full time equivalent (FTE) PC physician.[2] The relationship between patients and their PC providers should be "sustained partnership". In other words, a provider requires a manageable panel size in order to see patients when their demands increase, rather than postpone the appointment or bump them to another provider.[3] In order to actualize this relationship, managers in field of PC need to master the panel size management. A model to manage the panel size is in this part recommended. In other words, this model is used to define the denominator of physician to patient ratio when it is in form of 1:X (number of patients). An appropriately defined panel size improves patient satisfaction with healthcare; defines the workload; permits projection of patient's demand for healthcare; reveals provider performance issues; and helps

---

1. Murray et al. 2007, P. 45, 50
2. Murray et al. 2007, P. 45
3. Murray et al. 2007, P. 45-46

improve clinical outcomes.[1] Besides comprehending its importance, a manager should also know the methods to define both the current and target panel size as well as ways to make timely adjustments and improvements.

### 4.1.1 Defining the current panel size

It is simple for practices which are able to use health information system to define the panel size, as they could use electronic enrollment data of patients to capture the linkage between patients and physicians.[1] In Germany, people who have public health insurance are generally enrolled and codified in the German health information system. Since almost all of the German population is health insured by public insurers, using the enrollment data could be quite convenient in German healthcare organizations. In other environments, where patients are not codified in the information system, other approaches instead of utilizing enrollment data are always needed to link patients with physicians.[1]

The entire number of the unique patients who have seen any physician of a healthcare organization in the last 18 months is the current panel of this organization. This number is not difficult to define by using the enrollment data. Some organizations may tend to use data for the last 12 months. This may underestimate the current panel size, because many patients have no demand for physician services within a year.[2]

After figuring out the current panel size of a healthcare organization, the target panel size is easy to calculate. It equals to the current panel divided by the number of *clinical* FTE physicians in this organization. The entire number of FTE physicians subtracts the portion of each physician's nonclinical duties such as hospital rounds, operating room duties, management duties and meeting time is the number of FTE clinical physicians. For instance, a practice with 8,000 patients and four FTE clinical physicians would have a target panel of 2,000. Comparing the target panel size with individual physicians panel sizes could roughly judge whether a practice's workload is equitably distributed.[3] Because the individual panel size of a certain physician is often not identical with the target panel of

---

1. Murray et al. 2007, P. 45
2. Murray et al. 2007, P. 45-46
3. Murray et al. 2007, P. 46

23

his/her practice's, in the management it should also be defined. To determine it, we could directly use the patients enrollment data, who "belong" to him or her.

### 4.1.2 Determining the ideal panel size

Since the current panel size is not always the appropriate size, an ideal panel size must be defined as the gold standard in order to make timely adjustments and improvements. The ideal panel size is the result of a simple equation that quantifies the appointments demand and supply.[1] The simple equation:

> Ideal panel size × visits per patient per 18 months (demand) =
> physician visits per day × physician days per 18 months (supply).

The above equation can be used to define each physician's ideal panel size on the basis of his or her historical productivity. But it ignores quality of care or efficiency of resources usage and also does not take into account the delivery of physician visits by telemedicine or other new approaches. Thus it should not be used alone to define the ideal panel size of a physician.[2] Ideal panel size is not fixed, as it is determined by the three other variables in this equation. A practice may often prefer to raise the ideal panel size of a physician for different reasons such as expanding patients access to care, retaining current patients or increasing medical revenues.[3] But there's always a delicate blend of trying to increase the panel size of a physician with the panel a physician can give efficient, quality care.[4] Hence when changing the panel size of a physician, adequate and timely adjustments are also required from the following variables:

**Visits per patient per 18 months.** The average number of visits per patient per 18 months should be calculated by dividing the amount of unique patients seen in the last 18 months into the amount of visits to a practice that these patients create within this period.[5] When increasing the ideal panel size of a physician, the number of visits per patient per 18 months can be decreased by improving

---

1. Murray et al. 2007, P. 46-47
2. Muldoon et al. 2012, P. 31
3. Murray et al. 2007, P. 47
4. Hospitalist management advisor 2008, P. 1
5. Murray et al. 2007, P. 47

continuity, reducing rate of follow-up visits, prolonging the return visit interval, delivering more services per visit, using telemedicine such as e-mail and telephone care and new patterns of visits (e.g., group visits).[1]

**Physician visits per day.** This variable is not simply the number of planned appointments per day; it is determined by the historical data of number of visits provided per day. A practice could increase its supply of appointments per day by increasing the number of exam rooms, removing unnecessary work from the physicians, offering the physicians with more adequate help (e.g., advanced technology) and more "just in time" support so that they can reduce the length per visit.[2] These approaches could all help a practice to accommodate a larger panel.

**Physician days per 18 months.** This variable is the scheduled number of days a physician sees patients per 18 months. It can be affected by the illness of a physician, arrangement or organization changes within his/her practice, changing expectations about the number of days that should be scheduled for appointments, and rationalizing the distribution of a physician's time (e.g., replacing physicians away from nonclinical activities with clinical duties). A practice could sometimes be striking to observe that the amount of time physicians have contributed to appointment work is relatively or quite small, when analyzing this variable.[3] For example, one of the most prestigious ophthalmologist in Jiangsu province hospital serves outpatients only for about three hours weekly.

Analyzing these variables respectively could help healthcare organizations to understand how their operating patterns affect their panel size. The panel size is an outcome of the system in which physicians practice. The ideal panel size can be defined, but it should be necessarily adjusted in different circumstances according to all the healthcare provider and system factors.[4] The following worksheet can be applied to define the current and ideal panel size. It is a simplified model, since many complex factors such as physician support workforce (e.g., NPCs) are not taken into account.

1. Bodenheimer 2003, P. 797-798; Murray et al. 2007, P. 47; Schectman et al. 2005, P. 394;
2. Grumbach et al. 2004, P. 1247-1248; Murray et al. 2007, P. 48
3. Murray et al. 2007, P. 48
4. Murray et al. 2007, P. 49

**Exhibit 3.**

| | **PATIENT PANEL SIZE WORKSHEET** | | |
|---|---|---|---|
| | **Current panel** | **Example** | **Your practice** |
| A | The practice panel: The number of unique patients who have seen any physician in the practice in the last 18 months | 8,000 | |
| B | Full-time-equivalent (FTE) physicians | 5.0 | |
| C | FTE physicians devoted to non-visit work | 1.0 | |
| D | FTE clinical physicians (B - C) | 4.0 | |
| E | The "target" panel for each FTE clinical physician (A ÷ D) | 2,000 | |
| | **For an individual physician** | **Example** | **Your practice** |
| F | Clinical FTE of the individual physician being analyzed | 0.9 | |
| G | Actual panel for the individual physician | 2,000 | |
| H | Difference between actual and target panel for the individual physician (G-(E x F)) | 200 | |
| | **Ideal panel** | **Example** | **Your practice** |
| I | Visits per patient per 18 months | 3.19 | |
| J | Physician visits per day | 24.0 | |
| K | Physician days per year | 240.0 | |
| L | Ideal panel size ((J x K) ÷ I) | 1,806 | |
| M | Difference between actual and ideal panel for the individual physician (G - L) | 194 | |

Source: Murray et al. 2007, P. 47 and self-modification

The above model is particular suitable for an individual physician or practice (small-scale management). Certainly, it could also be customized according to some certain factors and conditions to manage the physician to patient ratio in large healthcare organizations.

### 4.1.3 Adjusting for age and gender

Age and gender can forecast appointment utilization and reflect patient acuity. Murray and others have collected appointment utilization data within a primary care practice over years. Patients were divided into 22 subgroups there based on age and gender. Every enrollment patient visits the practice about 3.19 times per year. The average number of visits per year in each age and gender subgroup was divided into the average visit rate (3.19) to define the likelihood of a visit within the subgroup. For instance, an one year old male is 3.28 times more likely to visit than a 55- to 59-year-old male, conversely a 5- to 9-year-old female is 1.60 times less likely to visit than a 70- to 74-year-old female.[1]

This data can be used to adjust physician's panel size, when a practice has sophisticated information system. Nevertheless, the adjusting procedure is complex and requires caution. For example, if a physician's panel of a practice is decreased because of higher acuity, panel sizes of other physicians within this practice must be

**Exhibit 4.**

Patients' likelihood of a visit, by age and gender

| Age | Relative weight | |
| | Male | Female |
| --- | --- | --- |
| 0-11 mos | 5.02 | 4.66 |
| 1 | 3.28 | 2.99 |
| 2 | 2.05 | 1.97 |
| 3 | 1.72 | 1.62 |
| 4 | 1.47 | 1.46 |
| 5-9 | 0.98 | 1.00 |
| 10-14 | 0.74 | 0.79 |
| 15-19 | 0.54 | 0.72 |
| 20-24 | 0.47 | 0.70 |
| 25-29 | 0.60 | 0.82 |
| 30-34 | 0.63 | 0.84 |
| 35-39 | 0.66 | 0.86 |
| 40-44 | 0.69 | 0.89 |
| 45-49 | 0.76 | 0.98 |
| 50-54 | 0.87 | 1.10 |
| 55-59 | 1.00 | 1.20 |
| 60-64 | 1.17 | 1.31 |
| 65-69 | 1.36 | 1.46 |
| 70-74 | 1.55 | 1.60 |
| 75-79 | 1.68 | 1.70 |
| 80-84 | 1.70 | 1.66 |
| 85+ | 1.57 | 1.39 |

source: Murray et al. 2007, P. 49

appropriately adjusted upward. Moreover, practices should utilize resources such as focused team support in order to manage the acuity factors more effectively, rather than only adjust the panel size.[1]

### 4.1.4 Adjusting for practice style

Healthcare policy-makers who wish to ensure every member of the population has a primary care physician may have a preference for larger panel size, while those

---

1. Murray et al. 2007, P. 49

advocating quality care may prefer smaller panels.[1] Physician with a highly personable style of practice may prefer conducting longer office visits, and thus could only warrant a smaller panel size. In a practice, where physicians are fix salaried, a physician with smaller panel size can be under discussion because he/she increases the workload of the other physicians. One possible solution is to adjust the physician's salary corresponding to the panel adjustment. For instance, a physician who practices with a highly personable style, resulting in a panel that is 90 percent the size of the typical panel in the practice, might be remunerated 10 percent less than a fully paneled physician of this practice.[2]

### 4.1.5 Ways to make improvements

A too large panel is harmful to continuity, since patients are often bumped to other providers. A too small panel is also a problem, since it won't bring enough revenue to support a healthcare organization. Strategies to decrease and increase the panel size without compromising quality of care are recommended in this part. Firstly, the strategies that reduce a physician's panel size:

- Let time attrite the panel size. Patients of a healthcare organization change insurance, move away or die every year.[3]
- Stop the over-paneled physician from enrolling new patients and seeing the patients of his or her absent colleagues, at least for a short term.[3]
- shift more resources to support the over-paneled physician. For instance, increasing the number of exam rooms, allotting (more) support staff (e.g., NPCs, clerical staff) to him or her.[3]
- Simply inform some certain patients of an over-panel that they have been moved to another physician within the practice or to a cooperated practice.[3]

These strategies could increase the physician to patient ratio of an individual physician, but might not change the overall ratio of a healthcare organization.

Secondly, the approaches that increase the panel size:

- Utilize alternatives to traditional visits.[4] For instance, providing group visits and telemedicine.

---

1. Muldoon et al. 2012, P. 28
2. Murray et al. 2007, P. 46
3. Murray et al. 2007, P. 50
4. Murray et al. 2007, P. 47-48

- Manage chronic disease by using the collaborated community resources.[1]
- Improve patient self-management.[1]
- "Ensure that all staff work to their full scope of practice."[1]
- Apply Advanced access model.[2]

The above strategies could not only decrease the physician to patient ratio of an individual healthcare provider but also the overall ratio of a healthcare organization.

## 4.2 Indirect management Methodology

Physician to patient ratio in large healthcare organization such as hospital and clinic should be managed indirectly. The working mechanism of indirect management methodology is matching the physician demand and supply by physician resource planning in order to generate the most appropriate physician to patient ratio possible "indirectly", and then improving it. The ways of generating and improving the physician to patient ratio are presented below.

### 4.2.1 Generating the physician to patient ratio

Physician to patient ratio could vary substantially by medical specialty. Hence an unified "gold standard" ratio of a healthcare organization can be nonsense for its single specialty. In other words, each specialty in a large healthcare organization should have their own physician to patient ratio. Missions to generate a right physician to patient ratio for each specialty in a healthcare organization can include configuring appropriate staffing level, defining the current demand for and supply of physician workforce, and improving the physician supply.

### 4.2.1.1 Configuring the appropriate staffing level

Right physician to patient ratio is crucial to running a cost-effective healthcare organization. Quality of care is also to consider when "creating" this ratio.[3] By configuring staffing level, the physician to patient ratio could be effectively

---

1. Muldoon et al. 2012, P. 30
2. Murray et al. 2009, P. 1042
3. Hospitalist management advisor 2008, P. 1

regulated. An appropriate staffing level does not overburden the physicians and allows them to achieve other professional pursuits.[1] The biggest value of it to healthcare organizations is the capability to improve efficiency and allow physicians to adequately handle their patients. If one of them could not happen, it's time to reconfigure it. Unfortunately, there is no simple answer for what the appropriate staffing level should be. Although many formulas are created to solve this difficult problem, none of them are really good, because the staffing level depends on what a healthcare organization can afford and what physicians it can get, which are difficult to determine scientifically.[2] Hence in order to be more efficient, every healthcare facility should consider all of its individual factors when defining the staffing levels and make the appropriate decision for their particular situation. Following objects must be examined, when attempting to define appropriate staffing level in a healthcare organization.

- Patient volume each day[1]
- Patient encounters each day (i.e., daily times that patients visit physicians)[2]
- Experience level of physicians[1]
- Utilization level of nonphysical care staff (e.g., midlevel providers, case managers)[1]
- professional expectations of physicians (e.g., engaging in advanced studies, publishing articles)[1]
- Requirements in specialty areas (e.g., more patients in ICU might require more physicians)[1]

**Patient volume examining**

Patient volume is the denominator of physician to patient ratio and thus one of its determinant. When patient volume increase (decrease), it is also sensible to drive the number of physicians upward (downward).[1] For instance, Physicians in Germany often work much less in July and August than in the other ten months because of summer vacations, thus to see a huge influx of patients in those two months. This aggregated patients load could be tough to handle and might force healthcare organizations to hire seasonal staff. Healthcare organizations without

---

1. Hospitalist management advisor 2008, P. 2
2. Hospitalist management advisor 2008, P. 3-4

part-time or seasonal physician options sometimes can suffer from understaffing during the peaks of patient load or overstaffing during the lulls. Hence healthcare organizations, which don't enjoy the flexibility of part-time or seasonal physician recruitment, should consider the seasonal fluctuations when configuring the staffing level.[1]

If a healthcare organization is running with a lower than appropriate physician to patient ratio, it might indicate that its patient load is excess. The excess patient volume could be the portent of potential revenue, a selling point for the administration of healthcare organizations. The administration should take advantage of the excess patient load to make extra revenue if a healthcare organization demonstrates its capability of handling its patients with high efficiency (quick admission of patients, treating them in high speed with high quality services, and discharging them without complications).[1]

**Experience level of physicians**

The level of physician experience is another consideration for configuring the right staffing level in healthcare organizations. The correlation between experience and efficiency is positive. Since the younger physicians are often less efficient in dealing with their daily work, it is suggested to build in extra time for them to improve when creating the right staffing mixture.[2] When younger physicians of a healthcare organization possess an obviously higher proportion among its entire physicians than before, and its overall number of physicians and patient volume are relative constant, it will make sense to increase the physician supply or shifting more resource to support the younger physicians. It is striking to observe that hospitalist who moves further away from his/her residency could develop an enhanced capability to multitask and over time. In this situation, they are able to see more patients a day.[2] This could mean good opportunities for younger physicians to improve their efficiencies. Healthcare organizations such as hospital chain should take advantage of this point when considering staffing levels.

Besides experience levels of the physician workforce, healthcare organizations should consider their individual program's overall specialties. The specializing

---

1. Hospitalist management advisor 2008, P. 2
2. Hospitalist management advisor 2008, P. 3

degree of a program alters the demand for physicians. For instance, physicians in surgery consulting programs could often see significantly more patients than their counterparts in programs that handle mostly new admissions, since the latter would spend more time with each patient.[1]

## Support

Healthcare organizations always have the absolute control over support staff that can be allotted to the physicians. Support staff such as NPCs (e.g., PAs or NPs), case managers, or administrative staff can all ease physicians' workload and thus increase their efficiency in patient care.[1] In the US, most hospitalists spend only approximately 35% of their time in seeing and treating the patients. Looking at labs and charts, at the nurse's stations, or writing notes cost the rest 65%. Anything could accelerate these processes will allow physicians to spend more time in handling their current patients or see more patients each day. Providing physicians with the best technology possible is a useful approach.[2] Advanced medical science and technology could sometimes reduce the demand for physicians that adequately treat a given population, and thus decrease the physician to patient ratio.

## Professional expectations of physicians

Nonclinical activities of physicians are driven by seniority, type of facility, and individual desires. Teaching, engaging in advanced studies or trainings, participating in committees and exploring other professional pursuits are typical physician's nonclinical duties. Physicians' working schedules should allow them to have enough time for that. This could always keep the physicians pleased in their careers and won't let them feel the necessary to leave for other ventures. Thus, healthcare organization wins a better overall physician attitude and retention rate.[1]

---

1. Hospitalist management advisor 2008, P. 3
2. Bureau of health professions et al. 2008, P. 52

## 4.2.1.2 Defining the current physician supply and demand

The current supply of the physician workforce of a specialty can be simply defined by checking the staff data, while determining the optimal number of physicians for a specialty is an imprecise science. An accurate definition of current physician demand could provide healthcare organizations with fundamental and reliable references to configure their staffing levels. Unfortunately, there's no simple formula for the number of physicians a healthcare organization needs to appropriately meet its staffing level.[1] However, several models and methods have been founded to define the current physician demand.

### Interviews/surveys

Medical staff often feels most comfortable communicating to their peers, since their expertise can be leveraged in the communication process. Consequently, physician interviews, medical staff surveys and focus groups could always have great implications on demand for physicians.[2]

### Physician supply/Demand instrument

By tracking ongoing changes in the current supply of physicians, a healthcare organization can roughly understand its "real time" physician demand.

### Physician requirements Model

After knowing some necessary information such as local demographic, payer and healthcare utilization statistics of market, a healthcare organization (e.g., hospital) can define the current (and future) physician demand for its individual specialties with the following model.

---

1. Hospitalist management advisor 2008, P. 1
2. Navigant consulting 2011, P. 2-3

## Exhibit 5. Physician demand model

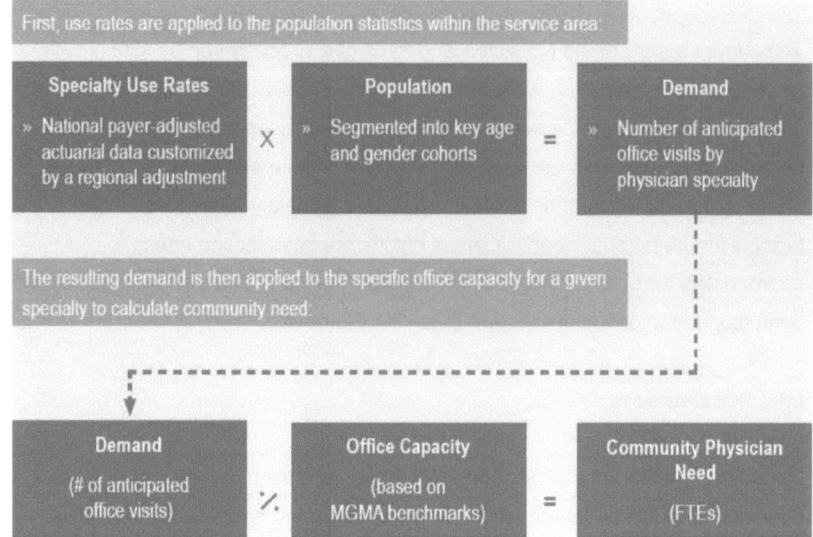

Note: MGMA= Medical Group Management Association (USA)
Source: Navigant consulting 2011, P. 2

## Benchmarking

To define physician demand of an object specialty, we could take the physician supply of its same specialty in another healthcare organization as the benchmark. The benchmark and target specialty must be in similar environments (e.g., demography, financial condition, level of medical technology). Two approaches are always used to chose the benchmark specialty. On the one hand, specialty that has relatively low numbers of physicians without any apparent compromise of patient welfare could be proposed as the current estimate of a reasonable physician workforce.[1] On the other, one would select specialties whose physician workforce maximizes efficiency while maintaining quality of care and patient access.[2] After being chosen, the benchmark should be customized in terms of the situation of each target specialty. Never apply it without adjustment.

1. Roos 1997, P. 1229
2. Fried 1997, P. 1227

### 4.2.1.3 Improving the physician supply

Jobs and candidates to fill them could often hardly match each other, which makes it tough to properly supply the physician demand, even if you know how many physicians you need to achieve the ideal staffing levels. Ensuring a large healthcare organization is adequately staffed is a universal challenge.[1] To complete this challenging mission, we should firstly recognize the physician supply status of each specialty in a healthcare organization (e.g., hospital). In other words, whether a specialty has physician shortage, adequacy or surplus must be defined at the beginning (the ways are already discussed in the first section). Afterwards, the work could be much easier.

### Resource reallocating

The medical resources within a healthcare organization can be mal-distributed at times. Shifting more physician support resources (e.g., physician, physician support staff, medical equipment) from the physician oversupply specialty to physician undersupply specialty is a useful approach. After the rational reallocation, if physician surplus still exists in some certain specialties, younger physician in these specialties could be sent to advanced studies, to another branch of a hospital chain (if they are in a hospital chain), or to rural or remote areas to help the physicians there. On the contrary, if some specialties continue to have physician shortage after the internal resource reallocation, following strategies can be effective.

### Staff Recruitment

Physician is a sort of resource that sometimes can easily outflow. Thus, before new physician recruitment, current physician workforce should be retained. Hire new physicians to supply the specialty, which is undergoing a physician shortage is a solution simply to think of. However, recruitment of new physicians is only one piece of the puzzle, sometimes it cannot completely solve the problem

---

1. Hospitalist management advisor 2008, P. 1

of a physician shortage.[1] Many other sorts of medical staff should also be hired at the same time.

Recruit more PAs, since they can carry out many of the normal physician duties. These duties can include preventive care counseling, performing physical exams, arranging for diagnostic tests, diagnosing, writing medical prescription, prescribing medical treatment, and much more.[2]

Recruit more NPs. "A nurse practitioner is a registered nurse that acquired additional education and training to carry out some of the tasks normally performed by a doctor." This can include, carrying out physical exams and screening, diagnosing, and treating illnesses and injuries (e.g., bandaging).[2]

**Excursus**

Facing physician undersupply, Jiangsu province hospital nearly do not recruit new physicians, because as the largest teaching hospital of Jiangsu province it has massive number of physician support staff to depend on. PhD, postgraduate students of human medicine, bachelor human medicine students who are in residency, and trainee nurses take large amount of tasks under the direction of the regular physicians or nurses of this hospital without salary. In mainland China, just like government agency, public hospitals are divided into different levels (i.e., province, city and district level). Younger physicians in hospitals of lower level are termly assigned to higher level hospitals to assist the physicians there (also without remuneration from the higher level hospitals). Hence they consist of another important portion of the physician support staff. The assist process is in fact advanced studies for them, because hospitals in higher level are always equipped with better infrastructure, more outstanding physicians and more advanced medical technology. In addition, lower level hospitals pay higher level hospitals for these studies rather than receive any revenue from the latter. Although utilizing these numerous support staff can save enormous costs for Jiangsu province hospital, differences between the support and regular stuff must be clearly recognized. Physician supply needs not only quantitative elements but also qualitative ones. In my opinion, relying on the physician support staff is

---

1. Navigant consulting 2011, P. 3
2. Noton 2009, w.p.

harmful for the development of a hospital.

## 4.2.2 Ways to improve the physician to patient ratio

After matching the physician demand and supply by physician resource planning, the physician to patient ratio could be already or nearly right. Many approaches can help a healthcare organization to improve it, several typical ones are stated as follows:

- Increasing the consistency of the physician schedules. For example, arrange physicians to work three or four days consecutively in favor of varying "off and on" days, as much resources (e.g., time, expense) can be wasted during physician transitions. In addition, a set schedule could lengthen the time that a physician sees and treats a particular patient.[1]
- Enhancing physician communication and communication between physician and the other staff when they are scheduled for their days off. This includes updating the staff about patients by using information technology such as email and websites.[1]
- Notify physicians of the benefits of implementing a consistent schedule when it applies to patient care. And engage the physician to come up with such a schedule.[1]
- Update the medicine and information technology in order to decrease physician's burden. For instance, computer orientated patient management can drastically save the time of non patient duties (e.g., patient files management), and thus increases the time that physicians focus on their patients.[1]
- Reducing a physician's time dealing with health insurers by simplifying business operations, since it can cost him/her many hours per day on the phone with their patients' health insurance providers. Establish a website that allows physicians to promptly capture the information about patients' covered treatments and procedures by their health insurance providers.[1]

It is significant to search for and implement methods to increase the physician to patient ratio, Since it will benefit the total medical care industry as well as the physicians and patients.[1]

---

1. Noton 2009, w.p.

## 5. Summary

"How many physicians are needed to adequately supply the patients demand for healthcare services" is the most important and difficult question to answer when managing the physician to patient ratio. "As many as possible in order to forbid poor consequences" is a right but glib and unpractical answer.[1] To make better answers healthcare organizations need guidance from health service researchers. Before the prescription is written, the changing and complex environment in which a healthcare organization operates must be understood. A physician to patient ratio may lead to acceptable healthcare outcomes in one setting but may cause problems in another.[1] Hence "one size fits all" ideal ratio does not exist. Every healthcare organization should have their accustomed physician to patient ratio. Otherwise, they could experience risky consequences related to equity, quality, efficiency of health service delivery and expenditure across themselves. Unfortunately, current strategies to define, adjust and improve the physician to patient ratio are fairly primitive, and many other factors add complexity to the ratio management missions. Further large-scale research work is needed to explore the relationship between physician to patient ratio and quality and efficiency of healthcare delivery, exam healthcare system factors that influence healthcare organizations and reduce medical spending.[1] In one word, much more evidence to guide us in answering the above question is urgently required.

---

1. Muldoon et al. 2012, P. 32

# 6. References

1. Bodenheimer, Thomas: Primary care in the United States. Innovations in primary care in the United States, in: British Medical Journal, Vol.326, 2003, P. 796-799.

2. Bureau of health professions/ Health resources and services administration/ U.S. department of health and human services: The physician workforce: projections and research into current issues affecting supply and demand, in: http://bhpr.hrsa.gov/healthworkforce/reports/physwfissues.pdf, from December 2008.

3. Cooper, Richard A. / Getzen, Thomas E./ McKee, Heather J./ Laud, Prakash: Economic and demographic trends signal an impending physician shortage. A new model of utilization, predicts an impending physician shortage, which the nation cannot afford to ignore, in: Health affairs, Vol. 21, No. 1, 2012, P. 140-154.

4. Council of state Governments: Physician shortages and the medically underserved, in: http://www.csg.org/knowledgecenter/docs/ TIA_Physician Shortage_Final_screen.pdf, from August 2008.

5. Dark, Cedric: The role of non-physician clinicians in primary care, in: http://www.kevinmd.com/blog/2011/07/role-nonphysician-clinicians-primary-care.html, from 22.07.2011.

6. Dill, Michael J./ Salsberg, Edward S.: The complexities of physician supply and demand: Projections through 2025, in: http://www.innovationlabs.com/pa_futur e/1/background_docs/AAMC%20Complexities%20of%physician%20demand,% 202008.pdf, from November 2008.

7. Fried, Bruce J.: Physician resource planning in an era of uncertainty and change, in: Canadian medical association, 157 (9), 1997, P. 1227-1230.

8. Getzen, Thomas E.: Forecasting health expenditures: short, medium, and long (long) term, in: Journal of health care finance, Spring, 2000, P. 56-72.

9. Grumbach, Kevin/ Bodenheimer, Thomas: Can health care teams improve primary care practice, in: The journal of the American medical association, Vol. 291, No. 10, 2004, P. 1246-1251.

10. Hospitalist management advisor: Finding the right ratio of physicians and patients is essential for efficiency, in: Hospitalist management advisor, Vol.4, No.7, 2008, P. 1-4.

11. Hospitalist management advisor: Patient-physician ratio affects Los, study says, in: Hospitalist management advisor, Vol. 4, No. 7, 2008, P. 6-8.

12. Institute of medicine of the national academies: Retooling for an aging America: building the health care workforce, in: http://www.iom.edu/~/media/Files/Report% 20Files/2008/Retooling-for-an-Aging-America-Building-the-Health-Care-Workforce/ReportBriefRetoolingforanAgingAmericaBuildingtheHealthCare Workforce.pdf, from April 2008.

13. Iroquois healthcare alliance: Physician shortage, in: http://www.workforcetv. com/ iroquois/IHA_PhysicianShortageProposal.pdf, from 2008.

14. Muldoon, Laura/ Dahrouge, Simone/ Russell, Grant/ Hogg, William/ Ward, Natalie: How many patients should a family physician have? Factors to consider in answering a deceptively simple question, in: Healthcare policy, Vol.7, No.4, 2012, P. 26-34.

15. Murray, Mark/ Davies Mike/ Boushon, Barbara: How many patients can one doctor manage, in: Family Practice Management, 14 (4), 2007, P. 44-51.

16. Navigant Consulting: Physician resource planning, in: http://www.navigant.com /~/media/WWW/site/downloads/healthcare/physician%20resource%planning. ashx/, from 2012.

17. New Jersey council of teaching hospitals: Economic impact of physician shortages in New Jersey, in: http://www.njcth.org/NJCTH/media/NJCTH-Media/pdfs/Econ-Impact-of-Physicians-in-NJ_nov-1_PEDSADULTS.dsbal.pdf, from 2010.

18. Noton, Adriana: Ways to improve the physician to patients ratio, in: http://talkbout.net/2009/11/18/ways-to-improve-the-physician-to-patient-ratio/, from 18.11.2009.

19. Riedemann, Niels C./ Kortgen, Andreas/ Reinhart, Konrad: Operative Intensivmedizin am Universitätsklinikum Jena, in: http://www.medicom.cc/medi com-de/inhalte/intensiv-news/entries/IN411/entries_sec/ Operative-Intensivmedizin-am-Universitaetsklinikum-Jena.php, from 2012.

20. Roos, Noralou P.: Physician resource planning: ways and means, in: Canadian medical association, 157 (9), 1997, P. 1229-1230.

21. Rürup-Kommission: Nachhaltigkeit in der Finanzierung der sozialen Sicherungssysteme, Bericht der Kommision, in: http://www.iwh-halle.de/d/abteil/arbm/Broschueren/Bundesministerium.pdf, from August 2003.

22. Salsberg, Edward/ Grover, Atul: Physician workforce shortages: implications and issues for academic health centers and policymakers, in: Academic medicine, Vol. 81, No. 9, 2006, P. 782-787.

23. Zurn, Pascal/ Poz, Mario Dal/ Stilwell, Barbara/ Adams, Orvill: Imbalances in the health workforce, in: http://www.who.int/hrh/documents/en/ imbalances_bri efing.pdf, from March 2002.